ORTHO

John Kingsley Walsh
MB, ChB (Otago), FRCSEd., FRACS (Orth).
Consultant Orthopaedic Surgeon

Published by John Walsh Ltd

© 2001 John Kingsley Walsh

First published in Great Britain in 1995 by John K. Walsh.
47 Alma Road, Windsor, Berkshire SL4 3HH

First published in 1995
Revised 2001

ISBN 0 9541409-0-7

Preface

I have on my bookshelf a book of 500 pages devoted to the front half of the foot, not even the whole foot. The literature in orthopaedics is immense.

I have printed this little book as a summary and a guide.

I have been greatly influenced by, and am largely indebted to, the late A. G. Apley, to whom I dedicate this book.

Acknowledgements
My thanks to Jo & Joe Design for their work on the illustrations and typesetting of this book

Contents

Foreword

Nicholas Andry, Professor of Medicine in Paris, devised the word Orthopaedia in 1741 as a title for a book that he wrote on the methods of preventing and correcting deformities in children. He devised the word from two Greek words, orthos meaning straight and pais meaning child.

The tree on the cover of this book is meant to denote that the child with splintage will grow straight, as will the tree.

This tree has become the symbol of every orthopaedic society throughout the English-speaking world. Orthopaedics itself has grown to include adults as well as children and is concerned with the musculo-skeletal system.

The patient, however, is a person who must be considered and treated as a whole.

A diagnosis must be established by following a plan before instituting appropriate treatment. Careful records must be kept both in hospital and in private practice.

DIAGNOSIS

Diagnosis is based on history, examination and investigations (*Symptoms, Signs, Tests*) :

SYMPTOMS : These are feelings experienced by the patient such as pain or stiffness.

PC	Present Complaints
HPI	History of Present Illness
FH	Family History
SH	Social History

SIGNS : These are findings on examination.

General Examination :

The patient is regarded as a whole; demeanour, dress, whether in pain, gait and attitude. The facial expressions and behaviour give a good guide to the underlying persona.

Local Examination :

Look	inspection
Feel	palpation
Move	percussion
Hear	auscultation

TERMS USED

1	**Supra- / Superior**	above
2	**Infra- / Inferior**	below
3	**Proximal**	towards the top
4	**Distal**	towards the bottom
5	**Medial**	on the inner side
6	**Lateral**	on the outer side
7	**Valgus**	away from the midline
8	**Varus**	towards the mid line
9	**Flexion**	bending forwards
10	**Extension**	bending backwards
11	**Abduction**	movement away from midline
12	**Adduction**	movement towards midline
13	**Pronation**	rotate inwards
14	**Supination**	rotate outwards

All joints at 0° in the erect position, except during 13 & 14
- elbow flexed at 90° thumb up is 0°

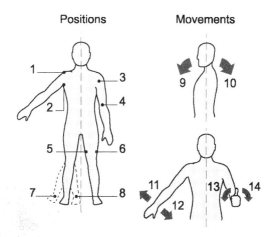

The body is divided into different systems:

CVS	Cardiovascular system
RS	Respiratory system
AS	Alimentary system
NS	Nervous system
MSS	Musculo-skeletal system
GUS	Genito-urinary system
LS	Lymphatic system
HS	Haemopoietic system

TESTS: If the diagnosis is in doubt or to confirm diagnosis tests are carried out; either on an outpatient or inpatient basis. They are expensive and should not be ordered indiscriminately or to anticipate the consultant asking for them.

X-ray AP (antero-posterior), lateral, oblique views are necessary to obtain the best information.

Blood Full blood screen to include red cell count, white cell count, ESR (the rate at which red cells drop in plasma).
Blood chemistry e.g. raised uric acid in gout
Blood culture if infection suspected

Urine Blood, protein, organisms, crystals

Sputum Culture, cytology

SPECIAL INVESTIGATIONS:

Computerised Axial Tomography (CT): Special X-Ray showing sections through the body.

Magnetic Resonance Imaging (MRI): Resonance of water molecules in a magnetic field shows soft tissues in vertical and horizontal planes.

Radio Isotope scanning: Uptake by bone of isotope shows hot or cold areas of increased or decreased bone activity

Contrast medium X-ray: Injection of radio-opaque material into a joint shows soft tissue

Arthroscopy: Looking into a joint

Arteriography: Injection of radio-opaque material into an artery measures blood flow through an area.

Bone mineral density: Tests whether bones have adequate calcium

Electromyography (EMG): Tests conductivity of nerves

Ultrasound : High frequency sound waves show soft tissues

Differential diagnosis is considered and an order of probability established.

Common things occur commonly.

EMBRYOLOGY, HISTOLOGY & PATHOLOGY

EMBRYOLOGY

The body develops from three types of tissue:

Ectoderm   Giving rise mainly to skin, but also to the nervous system.

Endoderm   This gives rise to the alimentary canal, its lining and the glandular structures that develop from it such as the liver and pancreas, also the respiratory and genito-urinary systems.

Mesoderm   This gives rise to the musculo-skeletal system.

6 Week old Embryo

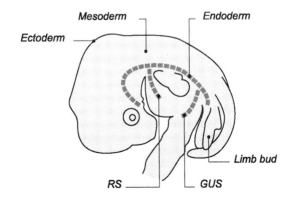

HISTOLOGY

The skeleton consists of bones articulated at joints. Bones are made up of a fibrous tissue set in calcium hydroxyapatite. Is it is the calcium which blocks X-Rays producing the shadow on the film. MRI (the resonance of hydrogen ions in a magnetic field) shows soft tissues well and is an excellent aid to diagnosis.

Long bones are hollow to provide lightness with strength. They are lined externally with a dense fibrous tissue called **periosteum**. This has the ability to make bone and is used to provide attachment to the muscles and tendons.

The hollow is filled with marrow, which is haemopoietic (producing red and white blood cells). In adults, the marrow is replaced by fat which in fractures may penetrate the vascular system producing a syndrome called fat embolism.

There are two types of bony tissue:

Compact bone: This is dense bone made up of Haversian systems with a lot of hydroxyapatite between the systems producing a dense appearance on X-ray.

Cancellous bone: This made up of bony trabeculae, usually aligned in the direction of force applied to the bone and which consists of thin plates of bone interspersed with haemopoietic tissue.

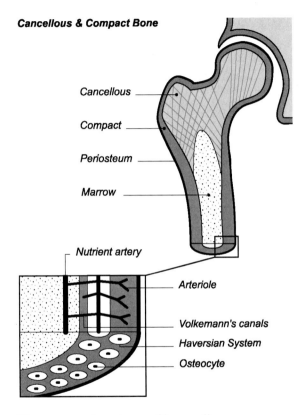

Cancellous & Compact Bone

Cancellous
Compact
Periosteum
Marrow

Nutrient artery
Arteriole
Volkemann's canals
Haversian System
Osteocyte

There are are three types of bone cell:

Osteoblasts These create bone.
Osteoclasts: These are giant cells which remove bone.
Osteocytes: These are adult bone cells.

Bony growth occurs at the ends of long bones at the Epiphysis, which is made up of cartilage cells multiplying, hypertrophing and calcifying and being replaced by bone cells (metaphysis). Remodelling occurs to ensure that the bone grows symmetrically. However, remodelling is also determined by the forces applied to the bone, the blood supply and nutritional supply; for example deficiency of vitamin D may produce rickets or bowing of the legs. Bone growth usually ceases at the end of adolescence but the last epiphysis to close is the inner end of the clavicle, around age twenty-four.

Growth Plate

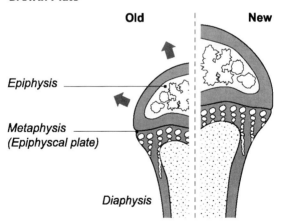

Bone requires a blood supply and is in a constant state of removal and replacement according to the stresses laid down upon it.

Bone reacts to stress or irritation by either:

1. Laying down bone due to overactivity of the osteoblasts, this first being described by Wolff where the amount of new bone laid down is in accordance to the force applied. Hardening of the bone is described as osteosclerosis.

OR

2. By loss of bone due to overactivity of the osteoclasts and this may be described as: osteoporosis (generalised loss, cystic formation (localised loss)

Sometimes a mixed situation may be seen, such as in some tumours or in Paget's disease.

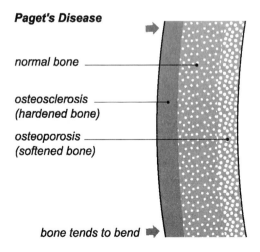

Paget's Disease

normal bone

osteosclerosis
(hardened bone)

osteoporosis
(softened bone)

bone tends to bend ➡

There are three types of cells in the body:

Labile: These are capable of reproduction and usually do reproduce all the time. They are usually derived from the ectoderm and endoderm such as skin and glandular tissue and the lining of the alimentary tract. Bone cells also fall into this category. These cells are the ones that usually respond to extraneous stimulae to become malignant.

Stable These cells such as the liver do not reproduce unless called upon to do so.

Permanent These cells lack the ability to reproduce and hyaline cartilage lining the joint is one type of cell. Nervous tissue cells and muscle cells also belong in this category. These cells rarely become malignant.

PATHOLOGY

Abnormal conditions affecting tissues gives rise to disease.

CONGENITAL: Faulty development in the embryo produces congenital disorders such as club feet.

ACQUIRED:

Inflammatory *(-itis)*. Acute / Chronic. Tissue reaction to irritation (e.g bacteria, chemicals) by the production of fluid and invasion of white cells and macrophages. Pus is this fluid and dead bacteria. A collection of pus is called an abscess. The suffix *-itis* is applied to the organ affected, such as tonsillitis, appendicitis.

2000 years ago, the Greek Celsus described the following as the effects of inflammation:

Rubor	redness
Dolor	pain
Calor	heat
Tumor	swelling

to which may be added **loss of function.**

Traumatic: This is injury to a tissue, the result depending on the force and the tissue to which it is applied. For example soft issue may be bruised or bone broken. Signs of inflammation are present. Bleeding into the tissues produces colour changes as the blood is broken down.

Neoplastic New growth of tissue independent of normal control (tumour).

Benign (-oma) This a tumour which remains localised

Osteo-chondroma

to an area. *-oma* is applied to the tissue affected such as lipoma - a fatty tumour, fibroma - a fibrous tumour. The effects produced depend on the situation. Swelling may be visible and pain may be produced from pressure on sensitive surrounding tissue.

Malignant **(-carcinoma, -sarcoma)** These tumours invade the surrounding tissue and metastatise to distant parts via lymphatics and blood stream. These secondary deposits are known as metastases or secondaries.

carcinoma:

Osteo-sarcoma

This usually applies to the tissues derived from the ectoderm and endoderm such as squamous cell carcinoma of the skin, adenocarcinoma of the breast, adenocarcinoma of the stomach. Early spread is to the lymph nodes and later via the blood stream.

sarcoma: This usually applies to tissues derived from the mesoderm such as fibrosarcoma, osteosarcoma, myosarcoma. Early spread is via the blood stream.

Effects depend on the rate of growth of the tumour and how quickly it spreads. Superficial tumours are more quickly diagnosed and treatment is often effective before they have spread.

Cancer is a word commonly used but is badly applied and creates fear, as not all malignant tumours are fatal.

Degenerative Ageing of the tissues. Such as spondy-
(-osis) losis meaning degeneration of the spine, arthrosis meaning degeneration of a joint (by common usage arthritis is the more used term).

Metabolic Diseases of metabolism. Affects the energy and the chemical processes in the body, such as gout, diabetes.

Endocrine Affects the glands, such as an overactive pituitary producing excess growth in children (gigantism) or in adults (acromegaly).

Immuno- Disorders of the immune system for
logical example, rheumatoid arthritis, AIDS.

Psycho- Where a person believes that there is a
somatic disorder when there is no organic cause, such as hysterical paralysis.

Iatrogenic Arising as a complication of medical treatment e.g. an injection causing nerve damage.

Idiopathic Unknown cause (usually blamed on a virus).

TREATMENT

Two words that summarise treatment are **kind** and **nous**. To be kind to someone means being gentle and treating them with courtesy and compassion. Nous means using one's commonsense and initiative.

Before treatment is commenced the prognosis or out-come of the condition must be considered as nature has a strong inbuilt mechanism towards healing and practitioners must assist nature as much as possible.

Results and complications (side effects) of treatment must be known . The cure should not be worse than the disease!

General
The patient must be treated as a whole person and includes not only the management of the acute situation but also convalescence and final recovery.

Local
Non-operative   (or conservative) This involves, for example, use of drugs, massage, manipulation and may be carried out by various disciplines.

Operative   (surgery) Pre and post-operative care are as as important as the oper-ation itself.

Various suffixes are used to denote operations:

- ostomy /	(cutting into) such as tracheostomy -
- otomy	(making a hole in the trachea), osteotomy (cutting into a bone).

- lysis	(freeing of) such as tenolysis (freeing of a tendon), neurolysis (freeing of a nerve).

- ectomy	(removal of) such as gastrectomy (removal of the stomach), appendicectomy (removal of the appendix).

- plasty	(refashioning) - such as arthroplasty (making a new joint), mammoplasty (refashioning a breast).

- scopy	(looking into) such as arthroscopy (looking into a joint), laparoscopy (looking into the abdomen).

Treatment involves a **team** which includes doctors, nurses, physiotherapists, occupational therapists, social workers, osteopaths, chiropractors and para-medical personnel and can take place either at home or in hospital.

A hospital is like a small city and efficient running requires the help of cooks, porters, engineers, telephonists, secretarial staff, cleaners, gardeners, and not least administrators.

There is pressure to minimise costs but this must not be allowed to minimise the quality of treatment although cost should be borne in mind.

Treatment is well exemplified by the following story.

My hero in medicine is Ambrose Paré who lived from 1510 to 1590. He was a French surgeon who spent 30 years in the army and later became a court physician . Late in his career he was sent by the King to look after Monsieur the Marquis d'Aurel who was dying as a result of a compound fracture of the thigh. He wrote in his journal:

I found him, in high fever, his eyes deep sunken, with a moribund and yellowish face, his tongue dry and parched, and the whole body wasted and lean, the voice low, as of a man very near death.

I found his thigh much inflamed, suppurating, and ulcerated, discharging a greenish and very offensive sanies. I probed it with a silver probe, wherewith I found a large cavity in the middle of the thigh and others round the knee; also several scales of bone, some loose, others not.

There was a large bedsore; he could rest neither day nor night; and had no appetite to eat, but very thirsty.

Seeing and considering all these great complications and the vital powers thus broken down, truly I was very sorry I had come to see him, because it seemed to me there was very little hope he could escape death. All the same, to give him courage and good hope, I told him I would soon set him on his legs, by the grace of God and the help of his physicians and surgeons.

Having seen him, I went for a walk in a garden, and prayed God to show me this grace, that he should recover, and to bless our hands and our mendicants to cure such a complication of disease. I turned in my mind what measures I must take to this end.

They called me to dinner. I came into the kitchen, and there I saw, taken out of a great pot, half a sheep, a quarter of veal, three great pieces of beef, two fowls, and a very large piece of bacon, with abundance of good herbs.

Then I said to myself that the broth of the pot would be full of juices and very nourishing.

After dinner, we began our conversation, all physicians and surgeons together, in the presence of Monsieur le Duc d'Ascot and some gentlemen who were with him.

I began to say to the surgeons that I was astonished that they had not made incisions in the patient's thigh, seeing that it was all suppurating, and the thick matter in it very foetid and offensive, showing that it had long been pent up there; and I had found with the probe caries of the bone, and scales of bone already loose.

They answered me, never would he consent to it; indeed, that it was near two months, since they had been able to get clean sheets on the bed, and that one scarce dared touch the coverlet so great was his pain.

Then I said, to cure him, we must touch something else than the coverlet of his bed. Each said what he thought of the malady of the patient, and in conclusion, they all held it hopeless.

I told them that there was still some hope, because he was young, and God and Nature sometimes do what seems to physicians and surgeons impossible.

I proposed free incisions for drainage, fomentations, a clean bed, hot water bottles, a pillow so adjusted as to relieve pressure on the bedsore, dusting powders, an opiate to ensure good sleep at night and a moderate allowance of wine. To help sleep artificial rain must be made, by pouring water from a height into a cauldron, so that it made the soothing sound of falling rain.

The diet should include raw eggs, plums stewed in wine and sugar, good broth from the pot, fowls and other roast meats easy to digest, good bread that was neither too stale nor too new.

Medicines prescribed must be properly flavoured, to disguise their taste.

This, my discourse was well approved by the physicians and surgeons. The consultation ended, and we went back to the patient, and I made three openings in his thigh. Two or three hours later, I got a bed made near his old one, with clean white sheets on it;

then a strong man put him into it and he was thankful to be taken out of his foul stinking bed.

Soon afterwards, he asked to sleep; which he did for nearly four hours; and everybody in the house began to feel happy, and especially his brother......

Then, when I saw him beginning to get well I told him that he must have viols and violins, and a buffoon to make him laugh; which he did.

In a month, we got him into a chair; and he had himself carried about his garden, and to the door of his Chateau, to watch people passing.

The villagers for two or three leagues round, now that they could see him, came on holidays to sing and dance, a regular crowd of light hearted country folk, rejoicing in his convalescence, all glad to see him, not without plenty of laughter and plenty of drink. He always gave them a hogshead of beer; and they all drank his health with a will.

In six weeks he began to stand a little on crutches, and to put on flesh and to get a good natural colour. He wanted to go to Beaumont, his brother's place; and was taken thither in a carrying chair, by eight men at a time.

And the peasants, in the villages through which we passed, when they knew it was Monsieur le Marquis, fought who should carry him, and insisted that he should drink with them; and it was only beer but they would have given him Hippocras, if there had been any, and all were glad to see him, and prayed God for him.

I tell this story to emphasise that kindness and common sense will often produce a cure; and Pare himself said "Je l'ai traité, Dieu l'a gueri"; (I treated him, God cured him).

It also shows the importance of accurate records.

CONGENITAL DISLOCATION OF THE HIP (CDH)

1/1000 live births (Female:Male 3:1)

Cause

It is thought to be due to laxity of the capsule of the hip, probably due to transfer of hormones across the placental barrier. Most babies have clicking hips at birth but only 1/1000 proceed to CDH. Pathological effects develop if the hip remains out of socket due to failure of development of the socket and head producing a shallow acetabulum and a small head of femur.

Diagnosis in Neonate

Ortolani Test : The hips are abducted with the knees flexed and a click or clunk can be felt and heard as the hip goes in and out of socket.

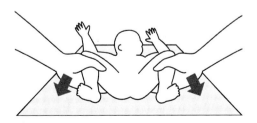

Ultrasound

X-Ray: Remember the ossific head does not appear before three months of age but the alignment of the shaft will show whether the head is dislocated (Perkins lines)

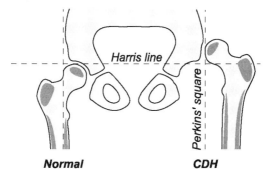

Normal   **CDH**

Treatment : The aim is to reduce the hip and hold it reduced to allow congruous development.

Early	a)	Maintain the hip in abduction Double nappies Pavlik harness Dennis Brown splints
	b)	Gallows traction with gradual abduction then hip spica cast

Late: If picked up late after walking (and the child is usually a late walker) treatment is not so successful.

 a) Closed reduction with adductor tenotomy
 b) Open reduction (infolded limbus)
 c) Alter acetabulum (Salter's osteotomy)
 d) Alter femur (adduction osteotomy)

Bilateral CDH should not be treated after four years of age, and unilateral CDH should not be treated after seven years of age, as complications of treatment may leave the child with more disability.

CONGENITAL TALIPES EQUINO VARUS (CTEV) (CLUB FOOT)
(Male:female - 2:1)

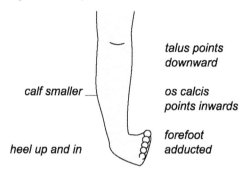

talus points downward

calf smaller

os calcis points inwards

forefoot adducted

heel up and in

Treatment : The aim is to get the foot plantigrade.

Early a) *Manipulative:*
Strapping / Splints / Plaster casts / Dennis Brown boots

b) *Operative:*
Difficult cases, which fail to respond within 3 months.
Soft tissue surgery:
Medial release / Posterior release Elongate TendoAchilles (ETA)

Late *Surgical:*
a) Calcaneo-cuboid fusion - (6-9y)
b) Triple arthrodesis: - sub-talar, talo-navicular, calcaneo-cuboid fusion (12-15 years)

CALCANEO-VALGUS
This is the reverse of club foot and is usually due to position in-utero.   Corrects spontaneously or with manipulative treatment.

FLAT FEET *(PRONATED FEET - PES PALNUS)*
Common - most require no treatment especially if the child has a good arch when standing on tip toes.

Treatment:
1.   Valgus insoles
2.   C & E (Crooked and Elongated) heels to shoes
3.   Surgery, if painful after growth ceases:
     • Advance tibialis posterior tendon
     • Fuse talonavicular joint

INTOEING
Common - usually due to increased internal rotation at the hips, often associated with the squatting (frog) position. Growth will usually correct this and reassurance to the parents is all that is needed. Sometimes it is necessary to apply C & E heels.

CURLY TOES
Mostly the third and fourth toes and most require no treatment but flexor tenotomy up to the age of four if under or over-riding adjacent toe.

GENU VALGUM / GENU VARUM
(KNOCK KNEES) / (BOW LEGS)

These are often found in early walkers (<1 year), due to unequal development of the tibial epiphysis. Most correct with growth and reassurance of the parents is all that is required.

Occasionally stapling of the epiphysis at the adolescent growth spurt or osteotomy after growth has ceased is necessary.

SPINA BIFIDA

Usually low lumbar spine with meningo-myelocoele (herniation of spinal cord and coverings) which may be open or closed and associated with paraplegia. Hydrocephalus (swelling of brain) associated.

Treatment:
1. Close defect
2. Treat paraplegia in infancy:
    muscle transfers or callipers
3. Urologist creates ileal bladder
4. Neurosurgeon performs shunts
5. Often the child spends first five years in hospital and becomes institutionalised, producing later problems.

CEREBRAL PALSY

1/1000 births

Brain damage from various causes, e.g. hypoxia, trauma, kernicterus (neonatal jaundice), infection. Usually normal or above average intelligence.

a) Spastic - tense muscles, scissor gait.
    Approximately 50%
b) Athetoid - writhing movements

Treatment
1. Splints
2. Muscle transfers or tenotomies
3. Education, better in normal school

MUSCLE DYSTROPHIES

These are rare and associated with genetic defects. Genetic counselling for the parents. Usually progressive and death from paralysis of respiratory muscles and associated infection.

ACHONDRODOPLASIA

Growth deficiency producing dwarf - usually normal intelligence

OSTEOGENESIS IMPERFECTA

Collagen disorder producing brittle bones, blue sclera.

Treatment:

1. Treat fractures as they occur.
2. Intramedullary rodding of femora and tibiae (kebab operation).
3. Genetic counselling.

OSTEOCHONDRITIS
Crushing, splitting and pulling

1. Crushing
The blood supply to a part is cut off (tissue necrosis). The dead bone erodes and is gradually replaced (creeping substitution).

	Perthes Disease (hip)
	(5-10, boys>girls)
Symptoms:	Pain, often in the knee. Limp
Signs:	"Irritable" hip. Decreased abduction of the hip
Tests:	Blood tests and X-Rays are often all normal initially. X-Ray change develop later with porosis and sclerosis, flattening of the head (mushroom effect) and in older patients the "sagging rope" sign.

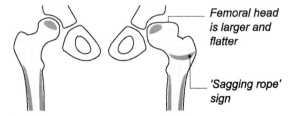

Femoral head is larger and flatter

'Sagging rope' sign

The effects depend on the amount of head of the femur involved and the age of onset. The earlier the onset and the smaller the amount of head involved the better the prognosis.

Treatment:

1.   Bed rest for the irritable hip for two to three weeks.

2.   Splint - weight relieving caliper, although this is now rarely used.

3.   Surgery - Innominate osteotomy to provide cover for the femoral head.

Scheurmann's disease (spine)
(12-17, boys>girls)

Symptoms: Backache usually in the thoracic spine.

Signs: Increased kyphosis (adolescent kyphosis)

Tests: X-Rays may show wedging of the vertebral bodies, Schmorl's nodes (disc intrusion into the bodies).

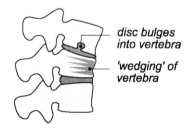

disc bulges into vertebra

'wedging' of vertebra

Treatment:

1.   Exercises
2.   Brace

2. Splitting   ***Dissecans :*** Part of the articular surface separates. Common in the knee (13-14, boys>girls)

Less common elbow, ankle.

Symptoms: Pain in the joint, clicking or locking

Signs: Often normal examination

Tests: X-Rays show separate fragment or loose body.

Treatment:

Arthroscopy and fix if possible with wires or screws, or excise

3. Pulling   Where a tendon pulls on an apophysis. Apophysitis.

Osgood-Schlatter's (knee)

(13-15, boys>girls)

Sever's (heel)

(9-13, girls>boys)

Symptoms: Pain

Signs: Local tenderness

Prominent tibial tubercle

Tests: X-Rays sometimes show a separate ossicle in the tibial apophysis, fragmentation of the calcaneal apophysis.

Treatment:

Most settle when growth ceases.

1. *Restrict activity :* Football in boys, ballet in girls
2. *Surgery :* Excise bony fragment.

SLIPPED EPIPHYSIS

Boys more than girls - 10-15, fat boys or tall and thin
40% bilateral; always X-Ray both hips.

      a)   Acute
      b)   Gradual

Symptoms: Pain in hip or knee.
                Limp
Signs: The hip goes into external rotation on
                flexion.
Tests: X-Ray shows disordered Trethowan's line,
                Shenton's arc, parrots beak (chronic)

Treatment:

                Reduce if possible. Internally fix.
                Beware chondrolysis and early onset
                osteoarthritis.

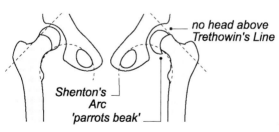

no head above Trethowin's Line

Shenton's Arc
'parrots beak'

Normal   **Slipped Epiphysis**

SCOLIOSIS

Deviation of the spine from the normal vertical alignment.

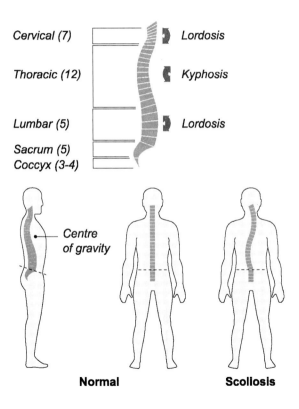

Cervical (7) — Lordosis

Thoracic (12) — Kyphosis

Lumbar (5) — Lordosis

Sacrum (5)
Coccyx (3-4)

Centre
of gravity

Normal   **Scoliosis**

Cause: Secondary to
a) neuromuscular disorders e.g. polio
b) infection e.g. T.B.
c) degeneration

Idiopathic
commonest; female >males; teenagers

Symptoms: Prominence of the back noted, often on
school examination.

Signs: Lateral deviation and rotation of spine
with rib hump on flexion (hunchback)

Tests: *X-Ray :* Standing views. Angle noted in
primary curve (Cobb).

Treatment:

Conservative:
a) Exercises
b) Splintage
• Milwaukee brace
• Risser jacket

Surgical: Curve > 40 degrees
a) Correction with rods (Harrington),
cables (Dwyer)
b) Spinal fusion

ACUTE OSTEOMYELITIS

Common in young children-organisms via the blood-stream to growing end of bone (metaphysis). Does not spread into the epiphysis due to adherence of periosteum and cartilaginous plate. May spread into diaphysis. Acute inflammation and pus formation follows. The pus is forced along the Volkman's canals producing subperiosteal spread along the shaft and around it. It may burst into the bone or out through the soft tissues. The commonest organism is Staphylococcus Aureus.

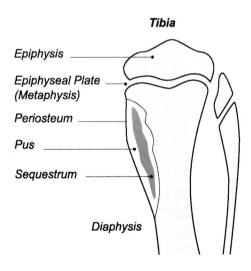

Tibia

Epiphysis

Epiphyseal Plate (Metaphysis)

Periosteum

Pus

Sequestrum

Diaphysis

Symptoms:	Child ill
	Acute pain
Signs:	Fever, septicaemia. Resists movement of joint, but movement possible. Compare joint infection, where no movement is possible.
Tests:	*Blood:* culture, full screen (raised ESR, white cell count).
	X-Ray: no change in early stages but later new bone formation beneath stripped periosteum.

Treatment:
Conservative:

    a)   Rest

    b)   Antibiotics - Penicillin and its derivatives, Methicillin, Flucloxacillin; Sodium fusidate

    c)   Splintage

Surgical:

    a)   Early drainage

Complications and results:

1. May go on to chronic osteomyelitis
2. Metastatic infection from septicaemia
3. Periostitis
4. Myositis

CHONIC OSTEOMYELITIS

Chronic inflammation usually due to sequestrum. This is an area of bone destroyed by acute infection, or loss of blood supply (common post surgery, for fracture treatment or joint replacement). This acts as an irritant producing further reaction and infection. Pus escapes through a sinus. Organism commonly MRSA (Methicillin Resistent Staphylococcus Aureus).

Symptoms:	Pain. Discharge.
Signs:	Skin thickened, red, scaly.
	Sinus present with discharge.
	Scars tethered to bone are evidence of previous bone infection.
Tests:	*X-Ray:* Bone thickened, with osteosclerosis and porosis present. Similar appearance in Paget's disease but bone bent.
	Culture: Organisms and sensitivity

Treatment:
Conservative:

    a)   Rest

    b)   Antibiotics

Surgical:

    a)   Drainage

    b)   Irrigation

    c)   Sequestrectomy, or removal of prosthesis.

    N.B. *Do not remove fixation until fracture united*

    d)   Saucerisation of bone

    e)   Occasionally amputation

ACUTE SEPTIC ARTHRITIS

Presentation similar to acue osteomyelitis - child resists movement of affected joint

Treatment:
1. Antibiotics Systemic and local into the joint
2. Drainage - essential early as raised intra joint pressure induces cartilage necrosis.

Complications:
Cartilage necrosis and development of stiff joint. More likely if infection becomes chronic.

POLIOMYELITIS

Common in underdeveloped countries. Virus affects anterior horn cells producing paralysis of various muscles. Preventable by oral or intradermal vaccination.

Balanced Paralysis: Flail

Unbalanced: Deformity

Muscle Strength:

0	Total paralysis
1	Flicker
2	Contraction but not strong enough to overcome gravity
3	Strong enough to overcome gravity
4	Strong but not normal
5	Normal

Child affected:

a)   Growth retarded

b)   Limb shortened and thin

c)   Vascular changes - atrophic skin

d)   Thin bones - causing fractures

Treatment
Conservative:

Splintage: Callipers, builtup shoe

Surgical:

a)   Leg lengthening

b)   Tendon transfers

c)   Joint fusion e.g. triple arthrodesis in foot

TUBERCULOSIS
Children (3-5) Adults
Infection with tubercle bacillus: lung, lymph nodes, bloodstream spread to bones and joints, caseous pus. Common in developing countries, and in migrants from them. BCG vaccination if high risk of infection.

General effects:	Night sweats
	Weight loss
Local effects:	*Joint:* Usually monarticular and large joint; Swollen. Associated muscle wasting. Stiffness
	Spine: Increased kyphosis (gibbus, kyphus)

Treatment
Conservative: Drugs:
- rifampicin
- isoniazid
- ethambutol
- streptomycin
- pyrazinamide

Surgical: Drain abscess, commonly called cold abscess (under anti-tuberculous cover). Synovectomy

Complications:
1. Fibrous ankylosis
2. Sinus formation and late scars
3. Late recurrence

FRACTURES AND DISLOCATIONS

Definition
1.   A fracture is a break in a bone
2.   A dislocation is a joint out of socket
3.   A subluxation is a joint partially out of socket
4.   A sprain is a stretching of ligaments

Fractures

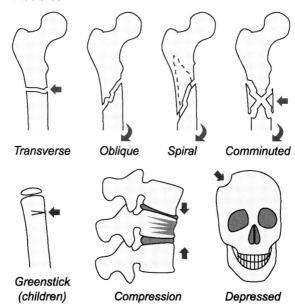

| *Transverse* | *Oblique* | *Spiral* | *Comminuted* |

| *Greenstick (children)* | *Compression* | *Depressed* |

Cause

A force applied either directly or indirectly. The degree of damage depends on the amount of force applied and the resilience of the bone. Pathological fractures occur with minimal force and indicate underlying disease, e.g. osteoporosis, secondaries. Stress fractures occur following repetitive minor force.

Types

1. Closed or open (skin perforated from with in or without - Gustilo classification).
2. Simple or complicated (involving vessel or nerve). Soft tissue damage is always associated and affects outcome.
3. Classified according to the appearence of the bone ends at the fracture site and this depends on the force applied (AO classification). Fracture description relates to the distal fragment (angulation, rotation etc).

Symptoms:	Pain. Loss of function
Signs:	Deformity
	Swelling
	Bruising
	Tenderness
	Movement at fracture site
Tests:	X-Ray
	MRI
	CT scan
	Ultrasound

Treatment:

Aim: Complete and early restoration of function. Before treatment can be considered it is important to know:

Site	Where the fracture is.
Type	The type of fracture
Displacement	Seen on X-Ray on 2 views, AP and lateral e.g. impacted, angulated, rotated. *Remember:* The description relates to the distal fragment.

General:

1. First aid and transport to hospital or surgery
2. Analgesia
3. Blood replacement if needed

Local:

Reduce   *Restore to correct alignment by:*

a)   Closed manipulation (the art of ortho-paedics - good bone setting)

b)   Open reduction (if closed impossible or inaccurate). Remember some fractures do not require reduction and a poor position in children can be accepted as growth will correct deformity (but not rotational deformity).

Hold   *If unstable or potentially unstable*

a)   External - Plaster, splintage, traction

b)   Internal - Screws, wires, pins, nails, plates. Beware devascularising bone.

c)   Combination - External fixateur, Ilizaroff. Useful in open fractures.

Use a)   Maintain and restore function.

b)   Exercise muscles and joints not immobilised.

HEALING OF FRACTURES

Healing is progressive and commences immediately. A good blood supply is essential for proper healing. It is conveniently divided into stages.

Haematoma : Bone bleeds and a clot forms between the broken ends. Bruising and swelling may be seen.

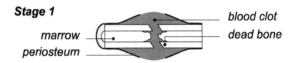

Stage 1

marrow
periosteum

blood clot
dead bone

Cellular proliferation : Fibroblasts, chondroblasts, osteoblasts and macrophages invade the haematoma over the succeeding 10 days.

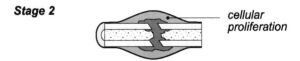

Stage 2

cellular proliferation

Callus : Woven bone is formed and calcification occurs over the next 4-6 weeks.

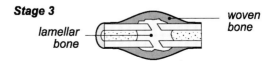

Stage 3

lamellar bone

woven bone

Consolidation : Lamella bone is formed and bone is laid down in lines of stress. This takes several months. Clinical union occurs during this phase.

Stage 4

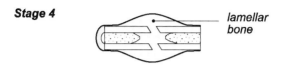

lamellar bone

Remodelling : The bone is restored as nearly as possible to the original and this process takes up to two years.

Stage 5

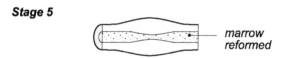

marrow reformed

Direct healing is seen in rigid internal fixation with no obvious callus. Indirect healing, where there is some movement at the fracture ends, shows callus.

Clinical union is defined when the bone is stable on examination. Radiological union when the fracture is consolidated on X-Ray.

Time *(half time for children)*

	Spiral fracture	*Transverse*
Upper limb	6 weeks	12 weeks
Lower limb	12 weeks	24 weeks

Factors affecting healing:

1.   Degree of local trauma
2.   Degree of bone loss
3.   Type of bone (compact, cancellous)
4.   Degree of stability
5.   Infection
6.   Involvement of joint (synovial fluid)
7.   Presence of local malignancy
8.   Radiation necrosis.

Complications:
General
1.   **Shock** *Hypovolaemia*
     Treat: fluid and blood replacement

2.   **Crush syndrome** *Fallen masonry*
     Muscles release acid myohaematin, renal failure.
     Treat: amputation, dialysis

3.   **Fat embolism**
     Long bone fracture; fatty acid pneumonitis
     Test: blood gases
     a)   *Hypoxia*
          • Tachypnoea
          • Tachycardia
          • Cerebral confusion
     b)   *Pyrexia*
          Treat : Oxygen, steroids

4.   **Deep Venous Thrombosis (DVT) and Pulmonary   Embolism**

    a)   ***Prophylaxis***
- Exercises
- Low molecular weight heparin (LMWH)

       Treat : Heparin, warfarin

Local

1.   **Bone**

    a)   ***Delayed union***: Poor blood supply, large gap, excessive movement

       Treat: • Bone graft
- Electrical stimulation
- Lithotrypsy

    b)   ***Non-union***

    c)   ***Mal-union:*** Inadequate   reduction or fixation. Can be accepted in some situations or treat by osteotomy.

    d)   ***Avascular necrosis:*** blood supply interrupted e.g. scaphoid, neck of femur

    e)   ***Osteoporosis*** due to disuse can lead to Sudek's atrophy, Reflex sympathetic dystrophy. Both painful and difficult to treat.

2. **Joint**

    a)   ***Stiffness*** : Commonest, usually due to prolonged immobilisation and lack of exercise of the joints not immobilised.
N.B. Instruct patients to move as much as possible joints not immobilised.

    b)   ***Osteoarthritis*** when joint surface is damaged.

3. **Soft Tissue Damage**

    a)   ***Nerves*** e.g. midshaft humeral fracture involving radial nerve.

    b)   ***Vessels*** e.g. popliteal artery in fractures at the knee.

    c)   ***Muscles***
- Wasting due to disuse
- Compartment syndrome
  Pain, pallor, paralysis, pulseless.
  Treat: Fasciotomy (emergency).
  Late result fibrosis (Volkmann's contracture - clawing of hand)

4. **Infection**

Commonly following open fractures or surgery
Treat • Antibiotics
       • Wound debridement

THE MANAGEMENT OF MAJOR ACCIDENTS

1. The management at scene and transport to hospital:
   a)   Establish airway
   b)   Protect spinal cord (hard collar, spinal board)
   c)   Arrest bleeding

2. Treatment in Casualty:
   ### *Primary survey:*
   A   Airway (c.spine control)
   B   Breathing and ventilation
   C   Circulation. Control haemorrhage Blood pressure, Pulse
   D   Disability (neurological status)
   E   Exposure (undress patient, keep warm)

   A   Alert
   V   Responds to vocal stimuli
   P   Responds to painful stimuli
   U   Unconscious

   R   Resuscitate

   ### *Secondary survey:*
   History
   Examination including Glasgow Coma Scale (GCS)
   Normal (15)   • Eye opening *(4)*
                  • Verbal response *(5)*
                  • Motor response *(6)*
   Repair damage - Priorities: ruptured spleen takes precedence over fractured femur.

FRACTURES AND DISLOCATIONS IN THE UPPER LIMB

Function is important: do not immobilise too long

Fractured clavicle : Very common. Union good. Figure 8 for 3 weeks or sling only. Warn mother of lump of callus in child.

Fractured scapula : Sling for a few days.

Fractured neck of humerus : Common. Elderly patients. Impacted fracture. Sling for 2 weeks under clothes then exercises.

Dislocated shoulder: Common anterior.

Reduce:	Kocher manoeuvre (traction, externally rotate, adduct, internally rotate). Hippocratic (foot in axilla, pull and adduct)
Hold:	Sling / body bandage 3-6 weeks
Use:	Exercises

Recurrent dislocation: Common, requires surgery, fix detached labrum (Putti Platt, Bankhart)

Fractured shaft humerus: Collar and cuff sling and gravity. POP splints

Supracondylar : Common in children.   Always admit; watch for arterial damage. Gross swelling. If necessary traction in extension. Mal union produces gunstock deformity.

Fractured neck & head of radius : Excise if comminuted. Exercise

Fractured olecranon: Gap fracture, reduce - hold by internal fixation

Dislocated elbow: Reduce. Stable. Sling for few days.

Fractured radius & ulna (both bones) : Difficult to hold, often best to operate.

Fractured radius & dislocated ulna :
at wrist - Galliazzi
Fractured ulna & dislocated radius :
at elbow - Monteggia
Always make sure both elbow and wrist joints are included in the X-Ray if there is a single bone fracture. Open reduction nearly always necessary.

Colles fracture :   Very common.
                        Fall on outstretched hand.

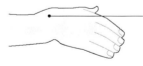
*Dinner Fork Deformity
(Radial deviation, dorsal
displacement, backward
angulation, comminution)*

Reduce: Traction on thumb and index finger, pronate, ventrally displace.
Hold: POP cast 4-6 weeks. Re X-Ray in 1 week as often redisplaces.
N.B. *Advise exercises. Shoulder, elbow and fingers.*

Smith's fracture / Barton's fracture: Reversed Colles. May require open reduction and fixation with buttress plate.

Fractured scaphoid: Common. Blood supply may be affected. If suspected (tender anatomical snuffbox) POP. cast, re X-Ray 1 week, 10 days. Cast 6-8 weeks, may require screw fixation.

Dislocation of wrist (lunate): Often missed. C.T. scan if unsure. Open reduction often necessary.

Fractured metacarpals: Usually no fixation. Exercise fingers.

Fractured base first metacarpal: (Bennett's fracture) Abduct thumb, may require open reduction.

Fractured neck fifth metacarpal: Boxer's fracture. Difficult to hold, not reduced, exercise fingers

Fractured phalanges: Strap to adjacent finger

Mallet finger: Rupture extensor tendon or base of distal phalanx Splint 6 weeks. Occasionally repair tendon

FRACTURES AND SPRAINS OF THE SPINE

Spinal injuries may be:
>   1. Stable
>   2. Unstable - beware cord damage

Mechanism of injury: Falls, Sport (rugby), Lifting,
>   Motor Vehicle accident (MVA), Falling
>   masonry (bombs, earthquakes).

Types:

1. *Extension* Chip fracture off anterior longitudinal
   ligament

2. *Flexion*   Crush or wedge compression fracture

3. *Compression* Straight spine, burst fracture

4. *Rotation*   Plus combination of flexion
   - unstable - may produce dislocation of
     facet joints.
   - unstable-cord at risk

STABLE FRACTURES AND SPRAINS

CERVICAL SPINE

1. **Soft tissue injury or muscular ligamentous sprain.**
Common following rear impact motor vehicle accidents. Whiplash is a term commonly used but it is more the mechanism of injury (flexion, extension jolt). Spondylosis (degeneration) renders the spine more susceptible.

2. **Wedge, crush or compression fractures.**

Symptoms:	Pain; neck, back of shoulder (trapezius) down arm (brachialgia)
	Headache
	Stiffness
Signs:	Restricted movements. Wry neck
Tests:	*X-Ray* - often normal or may show loss of lordosis in sprains. Wedge shaped vertibra in fractures.
	MRI - may show disc lesion but often present in normal population (about 20%)
	CT - in presence of fracture to determine if cord threatened.
	EMG - assess peripheral nerves in arm

Treatment:

General   a) Analgesics
              b) Anti-inflammatory drugs
              c) Relaxants

Local

              a) Collar- first two weeks
              b) Physiotherapy - traction, ultrasound, short wave diathermy, TENS machine (Transcutaneous Electrical Nerve Stimulation)
              c) Exercises
              d) Manipulation with or without anaesthetic
              e) Chiropractic
              f) Osteopathy
              g) Acupuncture
              h) Alternative therapy e.g. Aroma-therapy, Naturopathy, Reflexology

The majority of patients with neck sprains recover within 6 months (>80%), but recovery can take as long as 3 years, and 8-18% are left with permanent symptoms (usually older, with spondylosis). Studies have also shown no acceleration of spondylosis, or improvement after settlement of litigation.

THORACIC/LUMBAR SPINE

1. **Low back sprain**
Tissue injury, muscular ligamentous sprain, facet joint sprain. Usually after heavy lifting.
(Disc injury see Peripheral Nerve Lesions - page 74).

2. **Compression fracture**
Wedge, crush. Usually after fall, spontaneous in elderly osteoporotic women.

Symptoms:	Pain
	Stiffness
Signs:	Reduced movement, especially flexion
	Kyphus, Dowager hump.
Tests:	*X-Ray* - Loss of lordosis in sprains
	Wedging of anterior vertebra in fractures
	Generalised osteoporosis
	Osteolysis (metastatic deposit)
	Blood - Acid phosphatase if prostatic secondary suspected (raised). Alkaline phosphatase if lung, breast secondary suspected (raised).

Treatment
General: a) Bed rest
 b) Fracture boards
 c) Drugs; analgesics, anti inflammatories, relaxants.

Local: a) Corset, brace, plaster jacket
             b) Physiotherapy
             c) Exercises, swimming

Complications:
             a) Urinary retention
             b) Constipation
             c) Stiffness, may need manipulation.

SPONDYLOLYSIS

Defect in pas interarticularis. Often Asymptomatic
Tests: *X-Ray* - oblique scotty dog collar

'Scotty Dog' *(oblique view)*

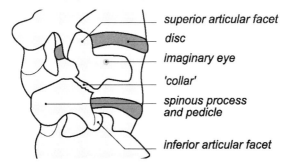

- superior articular facet
- disc
- imaginary eye
- 'collar'
- spinous process and pedicle
- inferior articular facet

SPONDYLOLISTHESIS

Grade 1-4 forward displacement of vertebra. May be asymptomatic. Back pain ± sciatica.
Treat :   Brace
              Spinal Fusion

UNSTABLE FRACTURES AND FRACTURE DISLOCATIONS

CERVICAL, THORACIC, LUMBAR SPINES
Immediate management important to end result
1. Transport to Spinal Injuries unit without delay
2. Take care to avoid further injury. Stabilise spine until properly assessed: Hard collar Spinal board
3. Maintain airway and ventilation

Cord damage
In 40 % cervical fractures, 5% thoracic / lumbar.
Lateral cervical spine X-Ray (all 7 and T1) mandatory in all patients sustaining an injury above the clavicle.
Signs: 1.   Spinal shock: • Loss of sensation
                                        • Loss of reflexes
          2.   Return of muscle function and spasms, rigidity (days to weeks later)

Quadriplegia: Paralysis all four limbs (Christopher Reeve, Superman)

Paraplegia: Paralysis lower limbs

Hemiplegia: Paralysis of one side of the body (due to cerebrovascular accident / stroke)

Treatment:
1. *Reduce*   open reduction if necessary
2. *Hold*   skull traction (Crutchfield tongs) spinal fusion

3. *Good nursing*

Essential. Applies to any patient especially elderly.

a) **Skin:** *Anaesthetic skin develops pressure sores within hours*
- No creases in sheets; no crumbs in bed.
- 2 hourly turning
- Wash and dry skin carefully
- Use powder and oil
- Adjust pillows
- Spinal beds - ripple mattresses
- Turning beds, moving patient helped if spine fused.

b) **Bladder:** *Avoid infection (ultimately leads to renal failure and death)*
- Catheterisation - strict asepsis
- Change weekly
- Antiseptics, antibiotics
- Train bladder by filling and emptying.

c) **Bowel:** *Avoid constipation*
- Train by aperients, enemas
- Abdominal exercises

d) **Muscles and joints:** *Avoid contractures*
- Physiotherapy
- Passive stretching

e) **Morale:** *Avoid depression*
- Role model (Christopher Reeve)
- Occupational therapy
- Special workshops
- Sports (Paralympics)

FRACTURES OF THE PELVIS

1. *PELVIC RING FRACTURES*
Displacement slight. Complications rare
Treatment: Rest, analgesics, mobilise when pain allows

2. *PELVIC RING DISRUPTIONS*
Displacement severe, large blood loss
Complications common:
a) genito-urinary tears
b) iliac vessel tears
Treatment:
Reduce: Traction, Open reduction and fixation
Repair : Soft tissue injury
Combined surgical approach depends on tissue damage

3. *AVULSION FRACTURES*
Treatment: Mobilise when comfortable

4. *SACROCOCCYGEAL INJURIES*
Coccydynia
Treatment:
Avoid sitting in acute phase
Ring cushion
Excise coccyx (coccygectomy), but results variable.

FRACTURES AND DISLOCATIONS IN LOWER LIMB

1. *FRACTURES IN FEMORAL NECK:*

    a) Subcapital (intracapsular)
       60-70 age group
    b) Inter-trochanteric (extracapsular)
       70-80 age group. More common in females
       as they outlive men.
    c) Sub-trochanteric

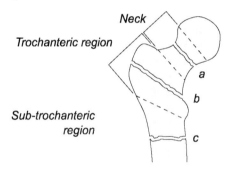

Signs a) Leg short
      b) Externally rotated
      Important queries as they affect length of stay
      a) Could patient walk before
      b) Home circumstances, Activities of Daily
        Living (ADL)
      c) Mental state

In general patient moves down i.e. If independent goes to live with relative; if there already goes to nursing home.

Treatment: Principles apply:

Reduce: All require operation,   fracture table. Often frail but operate as soon as possible.

Hold: a)   Subcapital, Garden type 1-4 (depends on displacement). 1,2 (mild) Internal fixation with compression screws.

3,4 (severe) Replace femoral head (Moore's, Thomson's prosthesis

b)   Inter-trochanteric, Dynamic Hip Screw (DHS)

c)   Subtrochanteric, Intramedullary rod e.g. Russell Taylor Nail.

Use: Commence walking as soon as possible.

Complications:

1.   Delayed union, non union.

2.   Avascular necrosis (30% Garden 3,4 therefore primary replacement).

3.   DVT and pulmonary embolism.

4.   50% of patients die within 2 years, because they are old.

2. *DISLOCATION OF HIP*

    a)   Posterior common, blow on knee. Hip flexed, leg adducted, internally rotated but beware concomitant fracture shaft when leg lies in external rotation.

    b)   Anterior. Leg abducted externally rotated

    c)   Medial. Fracture pelvis (floor of acetabulum)

Treatment:

Reduce: Under general anaesthetic by manipulation, or open.

Hold: By traction

Use: Exercise

3. *FEMORAL SHAFT FRACTURE*

1-2 litre blood loss, high, low

    a)   Transverse

    b)   Oblique

    c)   Comminuted

Treatment:

Conservative: Traction

    • Skin

    • Skeletal Pin through proximal tibia.

    • Ropes, pulleys and weights. Various: Perkins, Hamilton Russell, Thomas splint

Operative:

Intramedullary nailing under image intensifier control, with interlocking screws.

4. *FRACTURES INTO KNEE JOINT*

Aspirate haemarthrosis. Accurate reduction. Internal fixation. Beware popliteal artery damage;vascular surgeon on hand or transfer to centre with vascular unit.

5. *PATELLA FRACTURES*

a)   *Intact extensor mechanism (no gap).*
      Aspirate haemarthrosis, minimal support, active exercises.

b)   *Displaced.* Open reduction and tension band wiring. Patellectomy if comminuted (repair extensor quadraceps mechanism)

6. *LIGAMENT TEARS*

Medial, lateral, cruciates - increased "play", positive drawer sign. MRI helpful.

Treatment
Conservative:

a)   Aspirate haemarthrosis
b)   Cast or splint
c)   Physiotherapy

Surgical:

a)   Open repair medial or lateral
b)   Late reconstruction Anterior Cruciate Ligament (ACL).

7. *RECURRENT DISLOCATION PATELLA*

Common in teenage girls. Lateral dislocation (altered anatomical slope), lax ligaments.

Treatment

a)   Strengthen quadriceps.

b)   Realign patellar tendon.

8. *TIBIAL FRACTURES*

Proximal, middle, lower third

a)   Transverse

b)   Spiral or oblique

c)   Comminuted

d)   Fatigue (shin splints)

High ratio cortical bone therefore delayed, non-union likely. Beware compartment syndrome - Fasciotomy all four.

Treatment

Conservative:

Reduce: Manipulation under g.a.

Hold: Plaster or fibre cast.

Use: Crutches non or partial weight bearing (NWB, PWB).

Surgical: Elevation on Braun frame with calcaneal pin traction to reduce swelling for 2 weeks if comminuted and very swollen. Intramedullary nailing with proximal and distal locking screws. Reamed nailing promotes osteoblastic activity.

9. *ANKLE*

a) *Sprains.* Lateral ligament common. If total tear suspected stress inversion X-Ray. May require open repair.

Treatment: Ice

Strapping

Physiotherapy

b) *Fractures.* Inversion and eversion with rotation. Medial and/or lateral and/or posterior malleoli. Various classifications (used to be called Pott's fractures after Percival Pott who fell off his horse in1750 and broke his ankle. He spent his time recovering writing a treatise on fractures).

Treatment:
Conservative:

Reduce: Manipulation

Hold: Below knee cast 4-6 weeks

Use: Crutches

Surgical: Fix lateral side with plate and screws, medial, posterior with cancellous screws.

10. *FRACTURES OF TALUS/ CALCANEUS*

Fractures of the neck of the talus may jeopardise the blood supply and accurate reduction necessary.

Treatment:
Conservative:

- a) Ice
- b) Elevation
- c) Compression bandage
- d) Crutches, (NWB) 2 months

Surgical:

Arthrodese subtalar joint if pain persists

11. *FRACTURED METATARSALS*

a) *Base of fifth*	Common. Crepe bandage Crutches
b) *Neck third*	(March or stress fracture) Often noted on X-Ray with callus present

12. *FRACTURED TOES*

Aspirate subungual haematoma. Strap to adjacent toe.

PERIPHERAL NERVE LESIONS

Definition:

1.   **Neurotmesis:** Complete division

2.   **Axontmesis:** Incomplete division: intact sheath, disrupted axons.

3.   **Neuropraxia:** Intact nerve but doesn't work (physiological disruption).

Pathology:
Nerve is made of axons, cell safely in brain or cord

Division:
a)   Vascular and bleed-clot between ends
b)   Growth occurs from proximal end
c)   Distal end degenerates (Wallerian)
d)   Schwann cells (lining cells) grow in
e)   Axons regenerate,axons sprout
f)   Some may be obstructed : neuroma
g)   Growth 1-2 mm/day

Clinical features: depends on nerve
a)   Mixed: muscle wasting, skin numb
b)   Sensory: skin numb

Treatment:
1. ***Neurotmesis:***
a)   Repair nerve:
   • Immediate
   • Delayed (up to 4 weeks)
b)   Nerve graft: Gap too large - use operating microscope and fine materials (10 O nylon)
2. ***Axontmesis :*** Wait
3. ***Neuropraxia :*** Wait

Some injuries are difficult to treat e.g.
a)   Brachial plexus lesions
b)   Mixed nerves; median, sciatic
c)   Late treatment: Muscle transfers.

TENDON RUPTURES

1. ACHILLES TENDON
Sharp pain above heel. Gap palpable
Treat :   Repair - cast with foot in equinus
                (pointing down)

2. BICEPS TENDON
Characteristic lump in upper arm on stressing muscle.
May be preceded by pain due to tendonitis.
(There is a spelling mistake which persists in orthpaedic literature in which inflammation of tendons is called tendinitis).
Treat :   Repair not necessary

DISORDERS OF THE UPPER LIMB

1. *FROZEN SHOULDER (CAPSULITIS)*

Women>men, middle age. Pain and stiffness, later stiffness, gradual recovery

Treatment: Analgesics, anti-inflammatories
Local injection steroid
Physiotherapy
Manipulation (under g.a.)
Time: may take 2 years to recover.

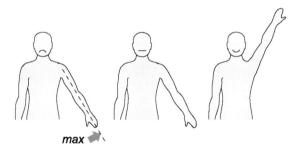

max

Initially *pain & stiffness*	*After 1 year* *stiffness only*	*After 2 years* *full recovery*

2.   *ROTATOR CUFF LESION*

Partial or complete tear of rotator cuff, usually supraspinatus. Painful arc of abduction or inability to abduct. MRI helpful. Calcification in tendon some-times seen.

Treatment
Conservative:

      a)   Injection local anaesthetic (l.a.) and long acting steroid,
      b)   Physiotherapy

Surgical:

      a)   Arthroscopy and repair
      b)   Sub acromial decompression
      c)   Latissimus dorsi transfer.

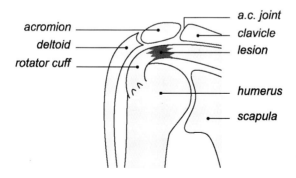

3. *LATERAL EPICONDYLITIS (Tennis elbow)*
and
4. *MEDIAL EPICONDYLITIS (Golfers elbow)*

Both are due to an irritation of the extensor and flexor origins, although uncommon in both tennis players and golfers!

Treatment
Conservative:

a)   Strapping
b)   Topical and systemic anti-inflammatories
c)   Injection l.a. and steroid.

Surgical:

a)   Release tendon and resuture

5. *REPETITIVE STRAIN INJURY (RSI)*

Painful forearm often in somewhat emotional young women and involving compensation claim, therefore not often believed, but real to the individual.

Treatment: Wrist supports
Change of work environment

6. *DE QUERVAIN'S TENOSYNOVITIS*

Inflammation of the extensor tendons at the wrist. Swelling, crepitus.

Treatment:
- a)   Topical and systemic anti-inflammatories
- b)   Injection l.a. and steroid
- c)   Release tendon sheath

7. *CARPAL TUNNEL*

Compression of median nerve at wrist - pain in hand (thumb, index, middle fingers) especially at night.

Treatment : Release flexor retinaculum.

8. *TRIGGER FINGER*

Swelling in the flexor tendon in the palm producing a "catch" or jerk as the finger is bent and straightened. Locked thumb in infants.

Treatment: Percutaneous or open division of the palmar pulley.

8. *DUPUYTREN'S CONTRACTURE*

Thickening and fibrosis of palmar fascia in hand affecting mainly little and ring fingers. Slowly progressive, pulling fingers into palm. Nodules in palm.

Treatment : Excise

MENISCAL LESIONS

1. *TEARS*

Medial > lateral, males > females (footballers), Bucket handle, anterior and posterior horn.

Cross-section of knee

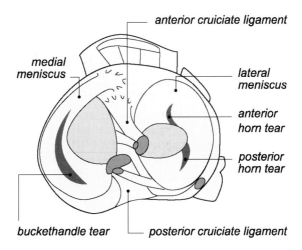

anterior cruiciate ligament

medial meniscus

lateral meniscus

anterior horn tear

posterior horn tear

buckethandle tear

posterior cruiciate ligament

Symptoms:	a)	Twisting injury
	b)	Pain
	c)	Swelling
	d)	Clicking and locking
Signs:		Click or clunk on McMurray test (rotation of flexed knee)
Tests:	a)	X-Ray negative
	b)	MRI

Treatment
Conservative:
- Quadriceps exercises
- Physiotherapy

Surgical:
- Arthroscopy, arthroscopic meniscectomy
  Late complication: Compartmental arthritis

ANTERIOR KNEE PAIN
Common in young females, often due to chondromalacia patella (softening of the lining cartilage).
Treatment
Conservative:
   a)   Restrict sporting activities
   b)   Physiotherapy

Surgery:
   a)   Arthroscopy and shaving patella
   b)   Realign patellar tendon

CRUCIATE LIGAMENT INJURIES

Rupture of the anterior cruciate (ACL) is common, posterior (PCL) uncommon, often associated with tear of medial ligament.

Symptoms:		Similar to meniscal lesions with a twisting injury.
Signs:	a)	Positive drawer sign, beware false positive in PCL where there is a backward sag.
	b)	Positive Lachman (leg is grasped firmly and moved relative to the thigh with knee bent).
	c)	Pivot shift (partial subluxation of tibia with knee bent).
Tests:	a)	MRI
	b)	Arthroscope

Treatment
Conservative:

a) Quadriceps drill (can often compensate)
b) Physiotherapy
c) Splint

Surgical:

a) Repair if acute
b) Reconstruct (late): Natural tendon (Patella, semitendinosis). Synthetic material. Allow 6 months to recover.

CERVICAL/LUMBAR DISC PROLAPSE

Anatomy: Disc made up of

a)   Central nucleus

b)   Outer lamellated annulus fibrosus.

Acts as shock absorber. If coating becomes worn, or put under abnormal stress nucleus may bulge through.

1.   Pressure on dura produces backache

2.   Pressure on nerve root produces sciatica

Intervertebral ligaments Anterior and posterior longitudinal.

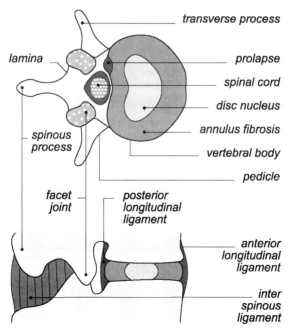

ACUTE

Symptoms:	Blow to head, sudden movement, heavy lifting or bending. *Pain:* neck, low back, down arm (brachialgia), leg (sciatica). Stiff spine (wry neck, cannot straighten up)
Signs:	Reduced movement especially extension Restricted straight leg raise (SLR) Muscle weakness Reduced or absent reflex Altered sensation Paraesthesia
Tests:	Plain X-Ray : loss of lordosis MRI (most helpful) CT scan, Myelogram, Discogram

Dermatomes   *Anterior*   *Posterior*

Treatment

Most patients recover without surgery

Conservative:

- Rest (bed rest 7-10days)
- Drugs:
    - Anti-inflammatory
    - Analgesics
    - Antispasmodics
- Local splintage
    - Collar, Corset or brace
- Traction
- Exercises
- Physiotherapy
- Chiropractic
- Osteopathy
- Acupuncture
- Chemonucleolysis

Surgical:

Indications

a) Failure of conservative treatment
b) Positive neurological signs (urgent if bladder dysfunction)
c) Positive lesion seen on MRI

Laminectomy and discectomy (microscopic). Spinal fusion if spine unstable.

CHRONIC / RECURRENT
CERVICAL/LUMBAR SPONDYLOSIS
(Low back syndrome)

Cause:		• Degenerate discs
		• Facet joint degeneration
		• Post traumatic scarring
		• Alternate pathology e.g rectal carcinoma invading sacrum
		• Aortic aneurysm
Symptoms:		Pain usually constant, deep nagging Radiation if nerve root involved
Signs		Reduced movement: Turning body to reverse car, difficulty bending to put on socks.
Tests:	*X-Ray:*	• Reduced disc space.
		• Osteophyte formation or lipping
		• Facet joint narrowing
		• Loss of lordosis
	MRI:	• Loss of water content of disc
		• Disc bulging
		• Spinal Stenosis (narrowing of canal)

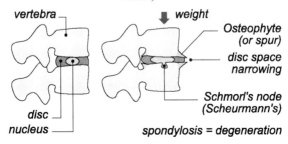

vertebra

weight

Osteophyte (or spur)

disc space narrowing

Schmorl's node (Scheurmann's)

disc

nucleus

spondylosis = degeneration

Treatment
Conservative:

>   Weight reduction
>   Exercise ; swimming, cycling
>   Drugs as for acute prolapse
>   Brace
>   Physiotherapy etc (as for acute)
>   TENS

Surgery:

>   Decompression laminectomy
>   Spinal fusion, anterior (neck)
>   posterior, intertransverse

Beware malingerers, especially in compensation cases

Signs: Restricted flexion of lumbar spine on standing but normal flexion on sitting up from the lying position.
Restricted SLR but can sit up with legs extended (equivalent to SLR 90). "Cog wheel" flexion of hips with knees bent.
Diminished sensation over the whole limb (glove and stocking) or even the whole side of the body.

AMPUTATIONS
Removal of part of the body

Indications:

1. Dead limb-gangrene from arteriosclerosis or severe trauma.
2. Lethal limb-may kill patient e.g. severe sepsis, malignant tumour.
3. Nuisance- too frail, stiff, or deformed.

Stump may be:

a) End bearing (weight through end of stump) e.g. through knee amputation. N.B. scar proximal.
b) Non end bearing (weight through soft tissues not end if stump) e.g.below knee amputation. Fish mouth scar.

Site of election:

Above Knee (AK) - 11 inches below great trochanter
Below Knee (BK) - 4.5 inches below tibial tubercle
Above Elbow (AE) - 8 inches below tip of acromium
Below Elbow (BE) - 7 inches below tip of olecranon

Technique:

1. Divide muscles, vessels (ligature), nerves (proximal), bone (bevel end).
2. Bandaging important

3.   Fit artificial limb:
- Immediate pylon, fibreglass
- Delayed

Below elbow amputation may be treated by separation of radius and ulna to give a pincer (Krukenberg operation)

Complications:

1.   Haemorrhage - leave tourniquet on the end of the bed.
2.   Skin problems with stump (scar too tight) - revise.
3.   Stump neuroma - excise more proximally
4.   Phantom limb - difficult to treat
5.   Exostosis - excise

HAND INJURIES
Principles of treatment

1.   Assess
2.   Fix fractures-usually internally
3.   Repair vessel and nerves
4.   Prevent swelling
- Elevate
- Cold pack or ice
5.   Maintain and restore function - exercise as soon as possible - MOST IMPORTANT

Definition: Mass of new tissue, which persists and grows independently of its surrounding structures. Often called tumours which really only means a swelling.

BENIGN Remains local, suffix *-oma.* Produces symptoms by pressure on surrounding tissue

BONE - Osteoma
- a) Ivory - lump on skull bones
- b) Osteoid - central lucent core
  Intense night pain relieved aspirin.
  Treat: Excision
- c) Cancellous - often cartilage capped.

CARTLIAGE- Chondroma
- a) Enchondroma inside bone, may cause pathological fracture.
- b) Ecchondroma, outside bone

BONE AND CARTILAGE- Osteochondroma
Bone capped with cartilage - Exostosis
- a) Single - Usually ends of long bones- points away from growth plate.
- b) Multiple- Diaphyseal aclasis - inherited 5% become malignant.

FIBROUS TISSUE - Fibroma.
Fibrous cortical defect. Fibrous dysplasia.
These rarely cause symptoms and show as defects on
X-Ray with cyst formation or sclerosis.

ANEURYSMAL BONE CYST
End of long bones - expansile - symptoms from pressure

UNICAMERAL BONE CYST
Children - ends of long bones (common-humerus)
May present with pathological fracture, due to
enlarged bone and thin cortex.
Treatment for both: Curette and bone graft.

HAEMANGIOMA
Rare - spine - backache- striated appearance on x-ray
Treatment: Radiotherapy

INTERMEDIATE
Locally invasive

OSTEOCLASTOMA
Giant cell tumour. Swelling at end of long bone usu-
ally in young adults, often painful.
Treatment: Curette and bone graft.
                    Radiotherapy

MALIGNANT

Invade surrounding tissue and metastatise via blood stream and lymphatics to produce secondary deposits.

PRIMARY TUMOURS
Rare

OSTEOSARCOMA
Young 10-20, old 5% Pagets disease, often end of long bones. Pain, swelling. Early spread by blood stream. X-ray Codmans triangle, sun ray.

Treatment: Amputation, radiotherapy, chemotherapy
                 <50% 5 year survival

CHONDROSARCOMA
Adults flat bones (scapula, pelvis) ends long bone metastatise late.

Treatment: Resection

FIBROSARCOMA
Often end femur, proximal tibia. Pain swelling.

Treatment: Amputate

EWING'S TUMOUR
10-20yrs, mid shaft commonly tibia Onion skin appearance on X-ray due to new bone formation as periosteum is lifted.

Treatment: Excise (amputate) chemotherapy

MULTIPLE MYELOMA

Middle age, pain, X-ray punched out "holes" in bones
Bence-Jones protein in urine.

Treatment: Local radiotherapy if practicable,
                Chemotherapy.

LEUKAEMIA

Ache in bones, fatigue (anaemia).

Treatment: Chemotherapy

SECONDARY TUMOURS (METASTASES)

These are the most common form of bone tumours,
and although carcinoma spreads mainly via the lymphatics blood stream spread to multiple sites in bones
is common in carcinoma of the :

    a)   breast
    b)   prostate
    c)   lung
    d)   kidney
    e)   thyroid

Bone pain, pathological fractures.

Treatment: Internally fix

CARE OF THE DYING PATIENT

    1.   Analgesia - do not withhold opiates
    2.   Good nursing - soft pillows and
          sheets, TLC (tender loving care)
    3.   Do not resuscitate - death is a release.

TUMOURS AND CYSTS OF SOFT TISSUES

Ganglion   Common wrist - jelly
Treat: aspirate or excise

Semimembranosis cyst
Behind knee - common in young boy
trans-illuminates. Excise

Bakers cyst   Behind knee synovial swelling associated arthritis no treatment.

Lipoma   Soft swelling in the subcutaneous tissues, reassure or excise.

Fibroma   Firmer lump

Neurofibromatosis
Multiple lumps in the skin, brown stains (café au lait), giant limbs (elephantiasis)

Neuroma   a) amputation - pain
Excise more proximally
b) Morton's - Pain, metatarsalgia, sole of foot usually 3-4 cleft between metatarsal heads.
Treat: metatarsal insoles, excise

Bursitis   Inflammatory swelling of bursa over bony prominences
a) Olecranon- drinkers elbow
b) Knee- housemaid's knee (pre-patellar bursitis)
Treat: anti-inflammatory drugs, excise.

The term arthritis should be reserved for inflammation of joints and arthrosis reserved for degeneration, but usage prevails. A joint is the place where bones meet and can be :

Synovial - Capable of movement, e.g. wrist, knees
Fibrous - e.g. symphysis pubis, distal tibio-fibular joint
Synostoses - e.g. joints of the skull

Synovial joints are affected by various disease processes:

                 Rheumatoid arthritis
                 Osteoarthritis
                 Gouty arthritis
                 Ankylosing spondylitis
                 Hallux rigidus, hallux valgus (bunions)

Synovial Joint

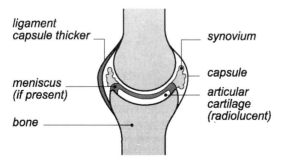

ligament
capsule thicker

synovium

capsule

meniscus
(if present)

articular
cartilage
(radiolucent)

bone

RHEUMATOID ARTHRITIS

1.   Aetiology: unknown, possibly auto-immune.
2.   20-40 female : male 3:1.
3.   Commences in the synovium: inflamed, thickened, (pannus), rheumatoid nodule, effusion.
4.   Gradually destroys articular cartilage - direct action.
5.   Ligaments become stretched, lax - deformity.
6.   Tendon sheaths affected - tendons may rupture (dropped fingers).
7.   Relapses and remissions occur - may burn out.

Symptoms: Pain one joint or several (polyarthritis)
            Malaise.
            Stiffness
Signs: Joints swollen, signs of inflammation.
            Commonly small joints of the hands.
            Synovial swelling and rheumatoid nodules
            Late: deformity Hands - MCP joints- Ulnar drift, dropped fingers (ruptured extensor tendons). IP joints Boutonniere, Swan neck
            Feet - Claw toes, bunions and hallux valgus
Tests: Blood • Raised ESR
                • Positive Rose Waaler and latex (75%)
                • Positive C reactive protein
        X-rays • Oseoporosis, Bone erosion
                • Joint space narrowing
                • Deformity

Treatment:
General

Drugs

a)   Analgesics, e.g. aspirin (also NSAIDS)

b)   NSAIDS (non steroidal anti-inflammatory drugs) inhibit cyclo-oxygenase (COX) the enzyme producing prostaglandins but also produces side effects such as gastric mucosal irritation.

c)   Anti-arthritic, Gold, Chloroquine

d)   Suppressant, Steroids e.g. prednisolone, long term side effects: Cushing's syndrome: thin skin with increased capillary fragility, bruises, osteoporosis, avascular necrosis (hip joint), obesity (moon face, buffalo hump).

e)   TNF - alpha blockers (tumor necrosis factor) eg. etanercept, infliximab.

Local

a)   Splintage - physiotherapy

b)   Synovectomy

c)   Salvage - arthroplasty

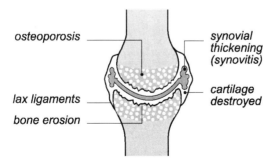

OSTEOARTHRITIS (OA)

Definition: Degeneration in a joint. The suffix *-osis* is used to denote degeneration but usage has prevailed to describe degeneration or wear and tear.

Cause and progression:

1.   Damage to articular cartilage - by trauma, faulty stresses, vascular problems, irritants (e.g. gout) producing Chondromalacia - softening and fibrillation of cartilage

2.   Damage to synovial lining - fibrosis of capsule, stretching and pain, gradually restricting movement.

3.   Damage to bone;
    • subchondral sclerosis
    • oteophyte formation, lipping
    • cysts

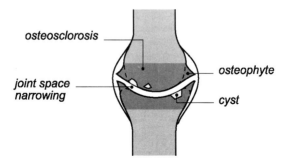

osteosclorosis

osteophyte

joint space narrowing

cyst

Symptoms: a) Pain

b) Deformity

c) Loss of function

d) Limp

e) Swelling

Signs: a) decreased range of movement

b) crepitus- grating on movement

c) limping- if in joints of the lower limb

d) Heberden's nodes in fingers

Tests: X-ray a) loss of joint space

b) sclerosis

c) Lipping or osteophyte formation

d) cysts

Causes of a limp from hip problems throughout life

0-3	C.D.H
3-5	T.B., Transient synovitis (irritable hip)
5-10	Perthe's
0-15	Slipped epiphysis
15-35	Trauma
35-50	OA secondary to preceding conditions
50+	Primary OA

Treatment
General:

a)   Rest - reduce activity, use walking stick

b)   Diet - reduce weight

c)   Drugs;

- Analgesics
- Anti-inflammatories (NSAIDS)

Local
Conservative:

    a)   heat

    b)   physiotherapy - ultrasound, exercises, shortwave diathermy, massage.

    c)   manipulation

    d)   built-up shoe

    e)   injections into joint

    f)   Arthroscopy and washout

Surgical

Osteotomy - surgical fracture to alter stresses through joint. Internal or external fixation.

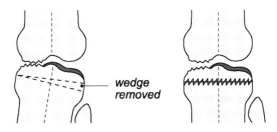

Arthroplasty - refashion a joint

a)   Create a gap to fill with scar tissue by removing part of the bone end (pseudarthrosis) e.g. Keller's procedure for OA of the big toe

b)   Replace one or both ends of the bone with prosthesis e.g total hip replacement (THR), total knee replacement (TKR).

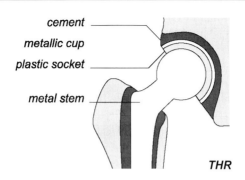

cement
metallic cup
plastic socket
metal stem

THR

Complications:
General

a) ***Blood loss - shock.*** Treat - blood replacement, may need to re-operate to find bleeding source

b) ***Deep vein thrombosis / pulmonary embolism.***

Prevent:
- Low molecular weight heparin/aspirin
- Elastic stockings (TED - thrombo embolic disease)
- Calf compression or foot compression pumps in theatre and after surgery

Symptoms: Calf pain, chest pain

Signs: Calf tenderness, pleural rub

Tests: Doppler
Venogram
VQ lung scan

Treatment: Anticoagulants - Heparin 10 days, Warfarin 3 months

Local

a) ***Dislocation***

Prevent: Abduction pillows in hip replacement

Treatment: Relocate - may need to reoperate and change alignment of (usually) socket.

b) ***Infection***

Prevent: Preoperative, operative and postoperative broad spectrum antibiotics.

Treatment: Antibiotics. Drain. May need exchange prosthesis - difficult. High risk of failure.

c) ***Loosening :*** a late complication usually after 10 years

Prevent: Compression cementing technique, hydoxyapatite coated prostheses in uncemented procedures.

Treatment: Revision difficult - operation twice as long as primary procedure. May need to convert to excision arthroplasty. (Girdlestone)

ARTHRODESIS

Bony fusion - Denude bone ends, insert cancellous bone, fix.

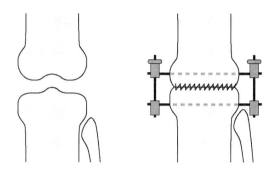

GOUT

1. Increased uric acid
2. Crystals in synovium: inflammation in joint
3 May damage cartilage and lead to OA

Treatment:

a) Drugs
   - Anti inflammatory
   - Allopurinol - decreased formation uric acid
   - Probenecid √ increased excretion by kidney
b) Surgery - as for Osteoarthritis

ANKYLOSING SPONDYLITIS

An inflammatory condition of the spine, progressive, males >females. Commences usually in the sacroiliac joints

Symptoms:	Pain, aching more than acute. Stiffness
Signs:	Local tenderness
	Decreased movement, loss of extension leading to a bent forward posture
Tests:	Blood - HLA antigen positive
	X-ray - sclerosis and bone loss in the sacroiliac joints. Bone formation in the apophyseal or facet joints of the spine, ossification of the discs leading to bamboo spine.

Treatment
Conservative:

> • Anti-inflammatory drugs
> • Physiotherapy - emphasis on exercise and posture

Surgical: Osteotomy of the spine if the bent forward posture is greater than 45°

HALLUX RIGIDUS , HALLUX VALGUS AND BUNIONS

Hallux rigidus is OA of the metatarso-phalangeal (MTP) joint of the big toe and pressure from osteophytes. Treat as for OA.

Hallux valgus is an outer sideways deviation of the big toe often associated with a medial or inner deviation of the metatarsal. An exostosis developes on the head of the metatarsal known as a bunion.

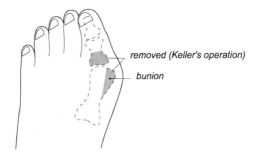

removed (Keller's operation)

bunion

Symptoms:	Pain from pressure of shoes
Signs:	Deviated toe, prominent bunion, reduced movement in the MTP joint in hallux rigidus with increased extension in the IP joint. Second toe often too long and forms hammer toe with fixed flexion of PIP joint.

Tests:	X-rays show medial deviation of the metatarsal and lateral deviation of the toe with an exostosis (bunion) on the medial side of the first metatarsal or osteophytes and joint space narrowing in hallux rigidus.

Treatment
Conservative:

Relieve pressure by   • Felt ring
                      • Hole in shoe
                      • Metatarsal bar

Surgical:

a)   remove bunion - exostectomy

b)   osteotomy metatarsal or proximal phalanx

c)   arthroplasty : exision (Kellers), replacement (silastic or titanium)

d)   arthrodesis-fusion (PIP 2nd toe)

PAGETS DISEASE

Named after Sir James Paget,

  1. Male>female 50-70 age group
  2. Cause unknown

Symptoms: Thickening of bone with osteoblastic and clastic activity- spongy soft bone.

Signs: 1. Pain
  2. Deformity
  3. Increasing hat size
  4. Bent bones
  5. Stress fractures

Tests: X-ray - Mixed osteoporotic and blastic activity. (see page 14)

Treatment
Conservative:

Drugs   • Analgesics
  • Fluoride
  • Biphosphonates

Surgical: • Osteotomy
  • Intramedullary rods for stress fractures in long bones
  • 5% malignant change.

VITAMIN DEFICIENCY

Vitamin D Rickets- soft bones especially distal tibia. Prevent with vitamin supplement

Vitamin C Scurvy- subperiosteal haemorrhage. Pain, loose teeth.

Treat - vitamin supplement.

(British sailors in the eighteenth century were known as limeys as they were provided with limes to prevent scurvy on long voyages)

OSTEOMALACIA

Loss of calcium from bone - malnutrition, post gastrectomy. Treat Calcium, vitamin D.

OSTEOPOROSIS

Loss of calcium as absorption greater than formation leads to decreased quantity of bone.

1. Postmenopausal
2. Disuse
3. Elderly

Pathological fractures common

Treatment : HRT (hormone replacement therapy)
Treat fractures as appropriate
No response to vitamin D

REFLEX SYMPATHETIC DYSTROPHY

This is an altered vascular response, often to minor trauma and leads to demineralisation of bone, changes in the skin and disabling pain which is difficult to treat. Spontaneous resolution can occur. Sympathectomy in some cases.

FIBROMYALGIA

Chronic pain syndrome but diagnosis still somewhat in dispute

Everyone has problems and sometimes people find relief from their problems through imaginary illness.

Placebo medication (no active ingredients) can provide relief in about 30% of cases, even with known diseases, such as duodenal ulcers.

Where a true psychotic state exists a diagnosis of conversion hysteria can be made. Treatment is extremely difficult.

The system of payment for injury may result in patients not wanting to get better from genuine injuries or feigning symptoms and signs (malingering), and the examining doctor for the court has to be as objective as possible.

Iatrogenic 8

Doctors are in a position where they can help many people return to health and most doctors enter the profession to do that.

However, sometimes mistakes happen e.g. prescribing a drug where there is a known allergy.

Negligence is accepted where a doctor goes beyond the standard of care considered by his peers to be reasonable.

As one teacher said to me "Know thy limitations" and I pass it on to you.

Summary

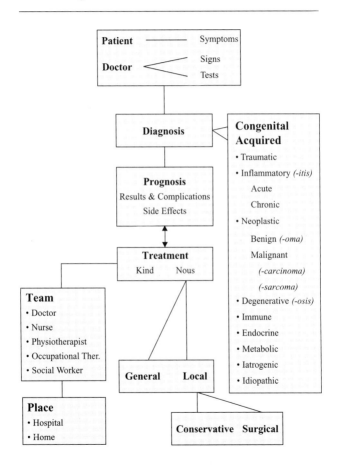

Index